Cognitive Behavioral Therapy

Techniques for Retraining Your Brain, Break Through Depression, Phobias, Anxiety, Intrusive Thoughts (Training Guide, Self-Help, Exercises)

I am grateful to my family for their help and support that was provided to me during the making of this little writing.

My father, wife and children dedicated.

P.S. You need to be patient, to go the way of healing with maximum efficiency.

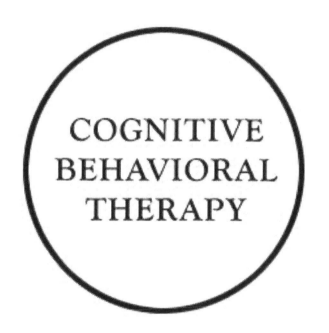

Copyright 2016 by Jack Oliver - All rights reserved.

This document is geared towards providing exact and reliable information in regards to the topic and issue covered. The publication is sold with the idea that the publisher is not required to render accounting, officially permitted, or otherwise, qualified services. If advice is necessary, legal or professional, a practiced individual in the profession should be ordered.

In no way is it legal to reproduce, duplicate, or transmit any part of this document in either electronic means or in printed format. Recording of this publication is strictly prohibited and any storage of this document is not allowed unless with written permission from the publisher. All rights reserved.

The information provided herein is stated to be truthful and consistent, in that any liability, in terms of inattention or otherwise, by any usage or abuse of any policies, processes, or directions contained within is the solitary and utter responsibility of the recipient reader. Under no circumstances will any legal responsibility or blame be held against the publisher for any reparation, damages, or monetary loss due to the information herein, either directly or indirectly.

Respective authors own all copyrights not held by the publisher. The information herein is offered for informational purposes solely, and is universal as so. The presentation of the information is without contract or any type of guarantee assurance.

The trademarks that are used are without any consent, and the publication of the trademark is without permission or backing by the trademark owner. All trademarks and brands within this book are for clarifying purposes only and are the owned by the owners themselves, not affiliated with this document.

CONTENT

Part I. – Introduction 6
   1. Cognitive-Behavioral Therapy 8
   2. History 10
   3. Theory 11

Part II – Variety of Cognitive Therapy 13
   1. Rational-Emotive Therapy 13
   2. Cognitive Therapy 14
   3. Training Self-Instruction 15
   4. Therapy Methods Hide Simulation 16
   5. Coping Skills Training 17
   6. Anxiety Control Training 18
   7. Treatment Methods of Solving Problems 19
   8. Resume 20

Part III – Cognitive Therapy of Aaron Beck 22
   1. The Methods of Cognitive Therapy 24
   2. Cognitive Therapy Technique 25

Part IV – Cognitive-Behavioral EXERCISES 27
   1. Anxiety Treatment: Cognitive-Behavioral Therapy 27
   2. Exercises to Overcome Fear 36
   3. Exercises to Relieve Stress 42
   4. Exercises Based on Techniques of Psych Synthesis, Assagioli developed 47
   5. Exercise Emergency Psychological Self-Help ("The mental dialogue with the mirror") 51
   6. Exercise for "Recharging Cyanogenic Dominant" (therapeutic and supportive exercise applied after the "coding"). 53

Conclusion 56
Author 57

Part I – Introduction

This book is the result of many years of research and clinical practice. Her appearance on the light is made possible through the efforts of many, many people - clinicians, researchers and patients. Paying tribute to the contribution of individuals, I suppose also, that in itself cognitive therapy is a reflection of the changes that have for many years taken place in the field of behavioral sciences and only took shape in the leading trend in recent years. However, we can not accurately assess the role played by the so-called "cognitive revolution in psychology" in the development of cognitive therapy.

Clinical observations, experimental and correlational studies, as well as ongoing attempts to explain the data, Contradictions of psychoanalytic theory led me to a complete rethinking of the psychopathology of depression and other neurological disorders. Finding that depressed patients do not have a need for suffering, I began to look for other explanations of their behavior that only "look" as the need for suffering. I wondered: how else can you explain their relentless self-flagellation, their steadily negative perception of reality and what seemed to be told about the presence of auto-hostility, namely their suicidal desires?

Remembering his experience of the "masochistic" dreams of depressed patients, which, in fact, was the starting point of my research, I began to look for alternative explanations for the fact that depressive dreamer constantly sees himself in the loser dream - he either loses some valuable thing, or It can not achieve some important goals, or appears defective, ugly, repulsive. Listening to how patients describe yourself and your experience, I noticed that they systematically reinterpreting the facts for the worse. These interpretations, shaped similar to the number of their dreams, made me think that depressed patients is inherent in a distorted perception of reality.

Thanks to several studies, we filled up our knowledge about how depressed patients evaluate their current expertise and its prospects. These experiments have shown that under certain conditions a series of successfully completed jobs can play a huge role in changing the patient's negative self-concept and thereby eliminate many symptoms of depression.

Cognitive therapy is constantly used in certain phases of the psychotherapeutic process in combination with other techniques. The cognitive approach to defects in the emotional sphere transforms the point of view of individuals to their own identity and problems. This type of therapy is convenient because it seamlessly blends with any psychotherapeutic approach orientation, is able to complement other methods and significantly enrich their effectiveness.

1. Cognitive-Behavioral Therapy (Cognitive Behavior Therapy)

Cognitive-Behavioral Therapy (**CBT**) - This approach is intended to change the mental images, thoughts and thinking patterns in order to help patients to overcome emotional and behavioral problems. It is based on the theory that behavior and emotions are partly due to cognition and cognitive processes, change that can be learned. Traditional methods of psychotherapy. Always recognized the important role of cognition in behavior and emotions, but cognitive behavioral therapy is different from the previous insight-oriented approaches in that it is only the material of cognition, there is a "here and now". Working with these cognitions held more systematically than in other methods of psychotherapy. It uses the principles of behavior modification to detect existing cognitions and identify those that are problematic. Behavioral techniques are used to eliminate unwanted cognitions, offers new thinking patterns and ways of thinking through issues and to support these new cognitions.

These techniques include:
a) registration of desirable and undesirable cognitions and fixing the conditions of their appearance;
b) modeling of new cognitions;
c) use of the imagination to visualize how new cognitions can be co-related with desirable behavior and emotional well-being;
g) The use of these new cognitions in practice in real situations, so that they become a common way of thinking of the patient.

Cognition, which change may be required, include separate opinions and beliefs and their systems, as well as thoughts and images.
Man organizes and uses of cognition by means of cognitive processes.

These processes include:

a) methods of evaluating and organizing information. about themselves and the environment;
b) information processing means. to fit in life and problem-solving, and c) methods of prediction and evaluation of future events.

2. History

Cognitive-behavioral therapy as an independent direction separated from the field of behavior modification and behavior therapy. Behavioral therapy 1960s. I tried to explain and treat emotional and behavioral problems by using the same laws of operant (et al.) of conditioning, which are successfully used in the study of the behavior of lower organisms, infants and those with mental retardation. However, it was found that even a very powerful external manipulation often could not change the natural behavior of the adult study. For example, in the treatment of depression can, in principle, support "happy" behaviors and punish "depressive". However, if the patient's cognitive processes include the tendency to self-incrimination or the vision of himself as a failure, the external manipulation will be ineffective.

Interest in self-control or the ability to independence from immediate rewards and punishments to achieve the objective contributed to the transition of many behaviorists from the concept of external control of behavior to theories postulating the possibility of using individual cognitive skills to solve problems in the environment. The thought process began to attach important role in determining the behavior and emotions.

Albert Bandura's monograph Principles of behavior modification ("behavior modification principles") has become an important event for many behavioral therapists who were in search of a more integrative model because it represented the theoretical interpretation of operant and classical conditioning, while stressing the importance of cognitive processes in the regulation of behavior.

3. Theory

Cognition is never addressed in the work with the lower animals. Human life is so complicated and we get through the voice channel so much information that cognition and cognitive processes can create something that is not an accurate reflection of the reality surrounding the individual. These cognitions can cause improper, unwanted behavior and / or emotions. The same environmental conditions may cause some people fear or depression and not cause any reactions in others.

People learn to meet their needs, observing the outcome of events and behaviors. On the basis of these observations they occur expectations about what will happen in the future and their own ability to act in such circumstances. They also show that a certain course of events causes certain emotional reactions. They compare themselves with others and form value judgments about their behavior and the behavior of others. Thus, our behavior is determined not only by external conditions, but also the decisions that we make on the basis of our cognitions about these conditions. So, cognition may cause unwanted behavior or emotions, depending on what the individual cognition learned to use in different situations. If people learn to think of themselves as losers, they may become depressed. If they start thinking that they can not cope with the situation, they will try to avoid it. The goal of cognitive therapy is to change the erroneous image of the patient's thinking about himself and his teaching skills necessary to deal with problematic situations. The therapy involves teaching experience, which aims to change the cognition of this, at once, to make them more appropriate and do not interfere with social or emotional development.

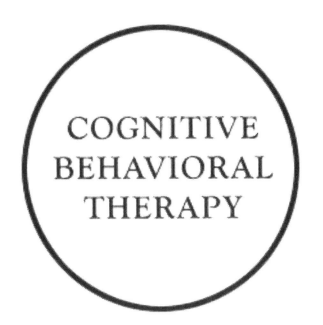

Part II – Variety of Cognitive Therapy

1. Rational-Emotive Therapy

Albert Ellis found in their patients the presence of irrational beliefs such as "I must be perfect" and "everyone should love me." These beliefs are accompanied by the concerns of the patient with the way people around him think about it. Any deviation from the reality of these beliefs the patient interprets as a terrible event. Because the reality rarely corresponds to irrational expectations of depression becomes probable. The therapy is based on the fact that patients are encouraged to adopt a more rational cognition by modeling appropriate thoughts. Patients are encouraged to monitor the quality of your thoughts, conscious registration frequency of their occurrence and impact on emotions.

2. Cognitive Therapy

A. Beck described how people can become depressed when they use distorted thinking. Examples of such thinking include fixation on failure rather than success, the belief that one failure is a total failure, and others. Cognitive tendency of seeing yourself in a negative light. Therapy consists in recognizing these trends and homework for production of successful experience. The patient demonstrate examples of more adaptive, positive cognitions, which he uses in practice as long as they do not replace old-style thinking.

3. Training Self-Instruction

D. Meichenbaum considered cognition as a self-instruction used in the development of behavioral skills. These instructions were at the level of consciousness in the early learning behavioral patterns. After the training instructions disappear from consciousness and behavior takes place automatically. Memorizing abnormal instructions may lead to undesirable behavior. If the instructions are incorrect or incomplete, the patient will experience anxiety due to the possibility of inadequate behavior. The therapy is to teach by modeling a new self-instruction. The patient, relying on your imagination, imagine using a new instruction system for the new behavior of the system. This therapy is used mainly with aggressive children and exam phobia.

4. Therapy Methods Hide Simulation

J. Kotel explored ways to teach people coping with stressful, anxiety-causing situations, offering them mentally rehearse the desired behavior. Patients learn to imagine what will happen as a result of their behavior and what actions they can take to deal with the situation. The patient also uses relaxation techniques. Thus, anxiety and stress do not prevent the implementation of the plan. This method was used in the treatment of phobias and self-doubt.

5. Coping Skills Training

This therapy is described M. Goldfridom, similar to the hidden modeling. The patient imagines a stressful situation, and then coping with anxiety. However, coping skills training (coping) imaging is performed in a series of increasingly frightening images. Using the technique of muscle relaxation allows you to carry a higher level of anxiety at each subsequent stage. Thus, the anxiety will never interfere with the patient to continue to work to improve coping behavior. It can also be practiced in role-playing problem situation. This therapy has been used in the treatment of phobias exams and helping people in coping with their own indecision.

6. Anxiety Control Training

This therapy is described by R. Sweeney and F. Richardson, it has similarities with other methods in the sense that it uses the mental representation of events that cause anxiety. The doctor teaches the patient to recognize the symptoms of anxiety and use as a signal for the use of coping strategies such as muscle relaxation or mental patterns, focused on success. This model is considered to be important to use a wide variety of imaginary situations, in order to better prepare the patient to a variety of real-life problems. It is commonly used with individuals who can not operate successfully in certain situations due to excessive anxiety.

7. Treatment Methods of Solving Problems

This kind of therapy is based on the fact that the resolution of the problems of life requires a set of cognitive skills such as the ability to select appropriate solutions means to obtain the expected results, to find alternative solutions and anticipate the results of these decisions correctly. In the absence of these abilities can arise behavioral and emotional problems. Under option behavioral therapy method for solving the problems developed Dzurilla T. and M. Goldfridom, patients are trained to clarify their problems, find possible solutions and best use of them. Patients register their own process mapping tools solutions and the expected results and the ability to evaluate their own behavior. This therapy has been used in the treatment of children with behavioral problems and adults with deficiency problem-solving skills.

M. Mahoney postulates that people are better able to adapt to life, if they are regularly used sequence of procedures for finding a solution like this, it makes a scientist or engineer. These procedures are:

a) specification of problems,
b) collection of information,
c) identification of the cause or the situational patterns,
d) analysis of options,
e) the restriction of the number of these options and their probing the,
f) a comparison,
g) the extension and revision of the options based on the results obtained.

8. Resume

The importance of mental processes as the possible causes of emotional and behavioral problems have long been recognized in all psychotherapy. approaches. However, the relationship between thinking, emotion and behavior is often attributed to abstract theories, making it difficult to understand their patients and empirical researchers estimate. In response to this bias in favor of the invisible and mysterious processes of behavioral therapy was limited only visible the external events. It was only later cognitive-behavioral therapy focused on thoughts as human behavior.

However, cognitive-behavioral therapy is not a return to the traditional insight therapy. In contrast to earlier approaches, cognitive behavioral therapy systematically explores the inner material, categorizing mental processes and linking them to external events in the careful observation of thoughts, feelings and behavior in the course of time.

Cognitive-behavioral therapy is aimed at training - through training - specific skills of direct relevance to the existing problem. In CBT the emphasis on the acquisition of skills and the patient's own responsibility for the results of the application of these skills can help improve the patient's self-control and ability to cope with difficulties. If in the end will be confirmed the effectiveness of cognitive-behavioral therapy as a treatment method, it will mean the successful application of the scientific method to the analysis and correction of our invisible thought processes.

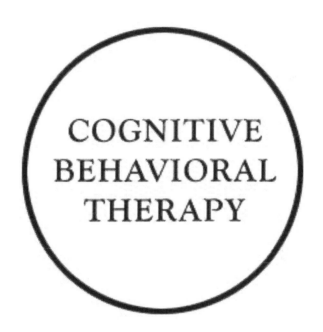

Part III – Cognitive Therapy of Aaron Beck

The term cognitive-behavioral therapy in modern psychiatry implies a whole range of methods. Each of them is based on the scientific belief that all possible violations in the psyche of any individual is the result of dysfunction of any view of the world and, consequently, violations of behavioral reactions.

First founder of this method, and the one who created the expected pattern of cognitive thinking, was Aaron Beck. It was he who in his work stressed the fact that the basis of psychological disorders and personality disorders may lie constant negative thinking. In his view, the perception of reality and its interpretation comes about in the next few stages: external stimuli affect the cognitive system which processes them in a certain way, creating a message, the result of which has already become a certain emotion, action, or a combination thereof.

On this basis, the scientist also suggested that people's thoughts cause a number of their emotions, the same. In turn, dictate the specific sequence of behavioral reactions, which subsequently have a place in society. Position Aaron Beck expressed as: "Not the world inherently bad, and people see it as such." If there is a dissonance between the inner world and interpretation of actual events taking place, and may develop a mental disorder. The basis of his works Beck put personal experience of observation and treatment of patients with neurotic depression.

During his research, he was able to identify three categories of thought, following which the individual is most often comes to the development of depressive disorders:

   a) Always predominant negative look at what is happening around. In other words, such individuals often have focused only on the negative aspects of any event or condition. While that life can provide them with exactly the same experience that brings pleasure to others but they are able to find in it only something bad and overwhelming.

b) Constant immersion in despair. The individual, thinking about your future, do not see it in perspective and any purpose. Such a condition stems from the previous one, but it deals specifically with the objective perception of the individual of their future, rather than taking place at the moment the event.

c) The same "negative attention" but aimed at its own "I". This condition is often called low self-esteem. Such individuals see themselves as weak, helpless, not independent, are not capable of anything.

He developed a system of cognitive therapy was based on this experience. It became a kind designed a method that is not only able to identify and highlight specific problems in the psyche, generating negative thinking, but also allows them to be transformed into the desired direction. Thus, cognitive therapy Beck still occupies a leading position among all the family and safe techniques in psychiatry.

Most often it requires no more than 30 sessions, which in time may not be too lengthy. In many ways, everything depends on the therapist. For example Aaron Beck himself suggested that physician-psychologist must appearance and judgments of the image to represent the standard to which the patient will seek.

1. The Methods of Cognitive Therapy

Today, developed and widely used many of the techniques of cognitive therapy. Of course, the most important of these are techniques aimed at combating the tendency to negative thinking, based on the change in the position of looking at things, rethinking of previous experience, a traumatic event from the past, childhood. It is also often used techniques based on imagination and self-suggestion by the patient. As a rule, the main objective is always forgetting the past and present negative experiences, and adherence to new beginnings.

Psychotherapy, based on such positions is aimed at suppressing the patient's desire for constant negative thinking, whether it is conscious or unconscious. This technique is most acute in the case when it comes to depressed patients. Such people, for example, at the recollection of past events can say that have forgotten how to be happy. When the therapist practicing cognitive therapy, it does not accept such statements without any comments.

From the point of view of the methodology, the expert encourages the reflection of the patient and his appeal to the past, but is trying to suppress thinking in a negative way. For example, in this situation, the patient can be asked about how to remember the situation when he felt happy and he gets overcome depression. In this direction, the main step is individual psychotherapy treatment to your inner "I", an objective assessment of their own judgment and discernment of the thoughts that are the cause of negative emotions.

2. Cognitive Therapy Technique

Such an approach in the treatment of compulsorily requires the formation of a cognitive mental status. This in turn is achieved by regular structured approach to learning, the creation of internal systems, training in the aspect of appropriate behavior.

The ultimate goal of the approach is to simplify the individual achievements of the following qualities:

a) The calculation of personal "negative" thoughts and reasoning.
b) Finding a permanent relationship between the type of your thinking, generated knowledge and experience and, of course, moving action.
c) Finding all the facts "for" and "against" certain pop-conscious settings.
d) Finding the most reasonable and appropriate explanation for the fact of their appearance.
e) Separate calculation of thoughts and beliefs that cause disruption of the inner self, as well as their transformation and "destruction".

As is clear, this approach allows time thinking in any situation to discover the way of thinking, which distorts and suppresses individual skills. Also, cognitive psychotherapy thinking can identify in a timely manner to allow suppressing thoughts, fear, or even prevent panic attack. Most often, an exercise in which the patient is able to achieve certain knowledge and skills include relaxation, ability to ignore and suppress the flow of thought.

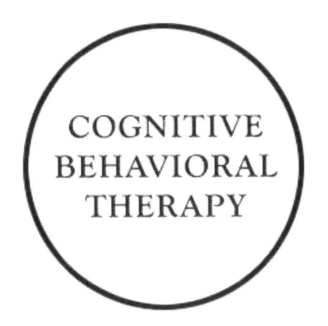

Part IV – Cognitive-Behavioral EXERCISES

1. Anxiety Treatment: Cognitive-Behavioral Therapy

This article discusses the main methods of treatment of anxiety. If you are prone to panic attacks or obsessive thoughts haunt you and unrelenting anxiety, this may indicate the presence of anxiety disorder. There is no need to live in fear and anxiety. In overcoming these problems can help the treatment, first of all therapy. Especially effective are its views as cognitive-behavioral therapy (cognitive behavioral therapy) and exposure therapy (exposure therapy). They will teach you to control the state of anxiety, restless thoughts and overcome fears.

Therapy will help to identify the underlying causes of your anxiety and fears, learn to relax, to see the situation in a new, less intimidating light, to develop problem-solving skills. Therapy gives you the tools to overcome anxiety and learn to use them.

Anxiety disorders are a few varieties. Therefore, to show you some kind of therapy. With obsessive-compulsive disorder (obsessional neurosis) treatment will be different than the panic attacks. The duration of treatment also depends on the type and severity of anxiety disorder. However, most types of therapy are not long-term. According to the American Psychological Association, many patients feel a significant improvement after 8 - 10 therapy sessions.

In the treatment of anxiety, there are different types of treatment, but the leading role is given to cognitive behavioral and exposure therapy. Each type of treatment can be used alone or in combination with other views. anxiety treatment may be individually or in a group of people with similar problems.

Cognitive-behavioral therapy (CBT) is the most widely used in the treatment of anxiety. Studies confirm its effectiveness in panic disorder, phobias, social anxiety and generalized anxiety syndrome, among other states.

- Cognitive therapy is studying the effect of negative thoughts, or cognitions, the state of anxiety.
- Behavioral therapy examines your behavior and reactions in situations where you experience anxiety.

The basic principle of cognitive-behavioral therapy is that no external circumstances and our thoughts determine what we feel at one time or another. In other words, the situation determines your feelings, and your understanding of this situation. For example, you are invited to the big gala event. You can come to different thoughts about this invitation, which will generate the corresponding emotion.

Situation: A friend invites you to a special event.

Thought # 1:

Festive event - it's fun. I love to go to parties and meet new people!
Emotions: You are happy and animated.

Thought # 2:

Parties - it's not my style. I would have rather stayed at home and watched a movie.
Emotions: Neutral

Thought # 3:

I never know what to say or do in front of other people. If you go and find myself in an awkward situation.
Emotions: Anxiety and sadness

As you can see, the same event triggers different emotions in different people. It all depends on the individual expectations, attitudes and beliefs. Negative thinking people with anxiety disorders cause negative emotions of anxiety and fear. The goal of cognitive behavioral therapy - to identify and correct negative thoughts and beliefs. The idea is that a change of thinking, you change the feeling.

Casts doubt on the validity of the previous thoughts in cognitive-behavioral therapy

Cognitive restructuring - it is the replacement of negative clichés of thinking that are of concern, the positive, realistic thoughts. It includes three stages:

1. Identification of negative thoughts. When anxiety disorder situation is more dangerous than it actually is. Take a person with a fear of germs, for example. For him to shake someone's hand - like death. Identify your fears is not so easy, even if you understand their irrationality. One method - ask yourself what you were thinking when we felt a sense of uneasiness.

2. Tucked questioning negative thoughts. In the second step should be to assess the thoughts that caused concern. You must analyze your negative beliefs, consider whether there is evidence of the truth of your fearful thoughts. Think are the chances that what you are afraid of, in fact, happen.

3. Replace negative thoughts realistic. Defining irrational assumptions and negative disturbances in your thoughts, you can replace them with true and positive. Make a realistic, calm statements that you will pronounce himself in the face, or in anticipation of a situation which usually causes anxiety in you.

Here's an example of how the process works replacing mental stamps in cognitive behavioral therapy:

Maria does not use the subway for fear of losing consciousness. Then, in her opinion, everyone will consider it abnormal. The psychologist asked her to write down your negative thoughts to determine erroneous or cognitive disorders and a more rational interpretation. The results are shown below.

Negative thought # 1: What if I lose my mind in the subway?

Cognitive Disorder: Waiting for the worst
A more realistic idea: I've never fainted before. It is unlikely that this will happen to me on the subway.

The negative idea # 2: If I lose my mind, this is terrible!

Cognitive Disorder: exaggeration, dramatization of events.
A more realistic idea: Even if I lose my mind, I'll be a few seconds. It's not so terrible.

Negative thought # 3: People find me abnormal.

Cognitive Disorder: to jump to conclusions that are not based on facts.
A more realistic idea: Most likely, people will worry if I'm okay.

Not so easy to replace negative thoughts more realistic. Negative thoughts often are long since formed stamps consciousness. It takes practice and time to break the habit. Therefore, in cognitive-behavioral therapy includes mandatory homework.

The systematic reduction of sensitivity to disturbing situations / objects

Exposure therapy is not shown to start with the big fears. This could injure the patient. Usually they start with a simple situation with a gradual increase levels of anxiety. Such a step by step approach is called systematic reduction in sensitivity to frightening situations / objects. This gradual desensitization allows step by step to improve self-confidence, acquire skills panic control.

Systemic desensitization includes three parts:

- Learning relaxation skills. Initially, the psychologist will teach you relaxation techniques, such as progressive muscle relaxation or deep breathing. When you learn how to counteract your fears, you will use this technique to reduce the physical reactions to anxiety, such as tremor or hyperventilation.

- Creating step list. Record 10 - 20 disturbing circumstances in order of their rise. For example, if you are afraid of flying, begin by viewing photos of flying planes, and at the end try the real flight. Every step you take must be clear and precise, and have a specific purpose.

- Work on tasks. The psychologist will help you go through all the steps established list. The aim is to be in a frightening situation for as long as your fears do not subside. Gradually you will come to understand that things are not as bad as you imagined in the mind. Each time with the appearance of disturbing sensations, switch to relaxation techniques. Relax, you can once again return to the situation. Your step by step efforts will certainly bring the final positive result.

Anxiety Treatment: Overcoming Fear of Flying

Step 1: Look at photos of planes
Step 2: Check out the video of the aircraft in flight
Step 3: Look at the rise of the aircraft
Step 4: Buy a plane ticket
Step 5: Pack items
Step 6: Go to the airport
Step 7: Sign up for your flight.
Step 8: Wait for landing
Step 9: You go in the plane
Step 10: Fly

Additional treatments for anxiety

You can also try additional methods of treatment of anxiety, which are aimed at reducing the general level of stress and achieving peace of mind.

- Physical exercise - it is a wonderful natural counterbalance to stress and unrest. Studies show that exercise three to five times a week lasting just 30 minutes will allow you to greatly improve your emotional state. The maximum effect is achieved with a daily hour of aerobic exercise.

- Relaxation techniques. Remarkable results are achieved with regular use of relaxation techniques such as meditation, progressive muscle relaxation, controlled breathing and visualization.

- Biofeedback. The use of sensors allows to control the physiological functions of the heart, breathing and muscle tension. Biofeedback shows your body's reaction to anxiety and gives you the ability to control them using relaxation techniques.

- Hypnosis. For the treatment of anxiety is sometimes used hypnosis. While you are in a state of deep relaxation, the hypnotherapist uses various therapeutic techniques to show you, what are your fears and teach you how to look at them differently.

If you find that have not used all my feelings or not realized some part of your body, repeat the exercise, focusing on the fact that you missed.

Every time you start to feel anxiety, perform this exercise stay in the present.

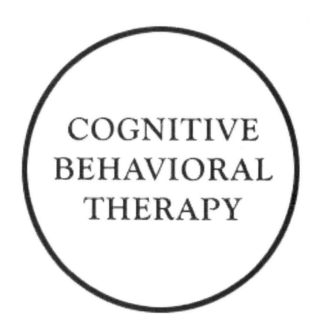

2. Exercises to Overcome Fear

If you are involved in an emergency, if you are in trouble and you have overcome fear, you can help a few tips to get rid of painful thoughts, thoughts and various fears associated with the situation.

Fear, as you know, is inherent in all animals, without exception, and people who in one way or another are exposed to various stresses, dangerous or emergency. But the fear and become your assistant in such situations, since triggered self-preservation instinct. But how not to succumb to the animal instinct to panic and learn how to control yourself and your own? What should be done and what your actions in the first moments of contact with the fear?

It is best to start with, do not succumb to it. And most importantly - do not give in to the strongest, "deferred to fear." In the first minutes, the fear is usually not so strong: he does not have time to learn quickly and completely human, it helps you resist the inertia of the previous state. But then, often after the disappearance of a specific threat, we have to seriously. But you can cope with that fear.

To do this, we must first learn how to switch easily, not "stuck" on the already over-past situations not "chew" them for too long, repeatedly returning to the same events. In addition, just ... do not be afraid. Especially do not be afraid, the probability of which is not so great. By the way, very often people, in contrast, can not be afraid of something to be feared.

One of the rules that normally helps to cope with fear - the ability to properly assess the reality and extent of the threat, as well as the opportunity to receive assistance. Never cover the eyes of fear - on the contrary, they try a little wider open and look around.

However, if you do not have coped with them, succumbed to fear and were temporarily "blinded", then try to quickly deal with it. It is useful to know at least the most simple psychological techniques.

For example, there is a most simple psychological trick: to feel fear: start slowly and breathe deeply: a deep breath - slow breath. Once again, even once more. And so at least ten times. Even if her purse snatched, and is far from the offender fled, it will help you quickly recover and raise the alarm. If the threat created is a different character (for example, it is not about to pull out her purse criminal, and requiring a ransom for your child terrorists), and developments are not so much fast, then this kind of "oxygen sedation" will have even greater meaning. This way you can effectively use the time available to fully adapt to the situation which has arisen to include in the work were stunned consciousness. And there, staring, awakened mind already he will come up with something useful.

Another very good reception is designed for more complex situation. Let's say that you were under the rubble in an explosion. Around the debris of concrete, and between them - a small niche, and in it - you. The situation is complicated, first of all - its uncertainty and instability. Succumb to panic, start to "twitch" in different directions - you start moving around the concrete slab, and the current relatively tolerant position has become unthinkable. Hence, it is necessary first of all to reassure themselves - so as not to make unnecessary involuntary movements.

For this very useful sometimes just to talk to himself, and calling several times by name. Talking with a useful in that it translates into an external plan interior often confusing experience - he had them as it unravels, builds into a coherent chain of cause-and-effect relationships, explains himself what happened, and in what position you were. Such a measured conversation with himself soothes, normalizes heart rate and other autonomic manifestations. Calling himself by name, you are referring to the childhood memory - it was in my childhood, we maximize protected, are safe, and that as a child they call us by name.

There is another useful technique. Think of a Woman Julia Description E. Izard: she was angry at the offender to snatch her handbag, and all the fear went somewhere.

Angered harder at something or someone: the situation for themselves and the other person. Anger replace fear, you will want to act immediately, and then you will no longer be afraid.

Fear can displace fear. Here is an example of a somewhat different scope, indicating the possibility of such effective displacement.

Example: A former military intelligence officer, was distinguished by his colleagues believe that "absolute fearlessness", told us that after the first stay among the enemy (in the role of one of them), he was afraid that one day may be exposed. "Once, when I was preparing for the next to throw the enemy territory, a feeling of uneasiness was particularly strong. Then I began to deliberately enhance it, assuring himself that I ever will definitely exposed and die. Napa feelings of fear, it was so strong that I kind of experienced in the thoughts and feelings of his own death. After that, I have no fear. Twice, when I was on the verge of failure, my equanimity embarrassed by my opponents and gave me time to get away from danger."

There are ways to Zen (Ch'an) training, leading, in particular, to the elimination of anxiety and self-control through the experience in the thoughts and feelings of his own death.

Techniques of this kind are quite complex and a great pleasure, but they are often quite effective.

Several ways how to overcome fear

1. The very first thing you must learn to do is to openly express their fear.

2. The next step in the fight against terror - is ... learn to be angry right. More precisely, to express anger and aggression. Here he writes about anger and aggression Everett Shostrom in his book "Anti-Carnegie or human manipulator." "Hatred - is frozen hostility. Hate - means to communicate their energy. In order not to destroy itself by hatred, it is necessary to pay in anger promotes contact ... ... Anger. Do you want to fight. The body tells it - frequent pulse and respiration, muscle tone increases. And the worst thing that you can do - is to suppress their physiological needs, to drive into the emotion. "

Now that the two most important areas (learn to show fear and learn to show anger) work with fear scheduled, you can talk about how to work with fear.

Exercises to overcome fear

1. Start with the acting technique: take facial expressions, posture is very frightened man - hide his shoulders, squeeze, bend your knees and try to feel or to restore the feelings experienced in a situation where fear. If the fear of aggression, remember this case, imagine yourself there again. Add a sense of fear. Yet! The more clearly you will feel fear, so much the better.

   Now, straighten your shoulders and take the pose of a happy man, smiling from ear to ear, laugh. You have to really feel the joy.

   Now become the aggressor - act out hatred, growl, hate. Now fear again, fuller, more clearly feel the fear. Now the

39

aggression again, this covering all the senses. Flows of emotion in the emotion. First, the transition will be slow. Then almost instantaneous.

2. Play with a partner, let him show you fear, and you show aggression. Then switch roles. If you do martial arts, try to play it in the ring.

3. Beat the other many and terrible as to be broken. Go to the boxing section. In shooting, this fear worked out shooting the photos that personally disgusts me, but shooting requires the destruction of the enemy, and it usually is needed in situations where there are several other rules.

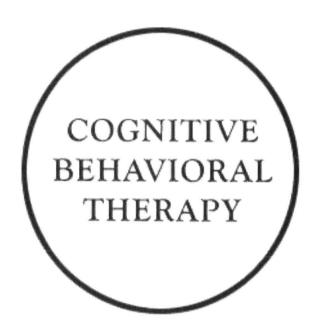

3. Exercises to Relieve Stress

All methods, sparing people from the effects of psychological stress, based on a single mechanism - the achievement of a particular psycho-physiological state, aimed at psychological relief (stress relief) and to switch brain dominant. To this end, we developed a variety of exercises, which are based is of psychoanalysis that helps achieve the state of harmonizing.

In today's dynamic life, stress is our constant companion. Life in a non-stop, filled with countless responsibilities and challenges that inevitably leads to tension and stress. Sometimes stress is a positive role - motivates us and helps us in the process of learning and acquiring new skills. However, most of all stress has a negative role on us - creates a constant feeling of anxiety and panic, provokes chronic fatigue syndrome, a negative impact on physical and mental health.

The search for effective methods for relaxation and exercise is crucial for a stable and happy life. Feel that stress disturbs the harmony of balance in your life? Then try to follow the recommendations below to relieve tension and stress.

With the help of the psychological impact on your body, you can restore emotional instability. To do this systematically perform relaxation exercises, preferably in the morning. Exercises allow after only a few days to feel the changes in the body: the acquisition of self-confidence, a burst of energy, increasing vitality and mood.

Exercise №1- "problem" - to relieve the emotional psychological state should find a problem that affected his appearance. After removing or dulling of the stimulus necessary to perform, the actions that help achieve inner peace: to be a comfortable position, relax, and imagine my side problem. An effective way in this situation is to compare the painful problem with global catastrophes worldwide, which will allow it to minimize;

Exercise №2- "inner light" - you need 5 minutes to relieve stress in this way. For this exercise, use the visualization technique, aimed at representation of a light beam that appears at the top of your head and slowly moving downward, illuminating the face, hands, shoulders, nice warm glow. Represent should not only light, but also its beneficial effects: the disappearance of wrinkles, the extinction voltage, charging the internal power;

Exercise №3- "mood" - helps to cope with stress after a quarrel over the 15 minutes. To perform the necessary pencils or markers by which you must present his state on paper, choosing appropriate colors and images. After drawing can express emotion words by writing them on the reverse side of the sheet. After graduating express their mood, "masterpiece" should break up, getting rid of negative emotions.

Win stress is not easy, especially alone. However, there is an opportunity to restore their emotional instability and strengthen the psychological state with the help of specially designed exercises and techniques aimed at combating and prevention against negative emotions.

7 simple exercises to relieve stress and nervous tension.

Gymnastics against stress.

1. Stretch the shoulders. Stand up straight and place your hands on his shoulders. At that moment, when you breathe in, lift the elbows hands as high as possible, and tilt your head back. On the exhale, return to starting position. Repeat this exercise several times to relieve tension in the neck, shoulders and back.

2. Reach for the stars. Stand with your feet shoulder width apart. During inhalation, stretch your arms up and stretch as if you are trying to reach the stars. On the

exhale, let go and shake hands, take a starting position. Repeat 5 times. For greater effect on the exercise, try to breathe deeply and spread wide his fingers in that moment, when you drag to the top.

3. Foot Girth. Sit up straight in a chair without wheels. Push the legs to him so that his toes were on the edge of his chair, and his chin was between his knees. Clasp your hands and feet very much to push yourself. In this position, you need to spend about ten seconds, and then abruptly loosen his grip. Repeat this exercise 5 times. This exercise will relax the muscles of the back and shoulders. Exercise is recommended to do in the morning after a heavy night out or a long sleep, if you feel the weakness in the muscles.

4. Child Pose. Sit on your heels and bare knees outward. During a deep breath and put your hands up a little stretch. Then exhale already put his hands to his knees, and then on the floor in front of you as far as possible and hold in this position 30 seconds Try to breathe in this position deeply and evenly. Return to starting position, repeat this exercise 5 times.

Breathing exercises to relieve stress

5. The slow inhale and exhale. To breathe in slow start, assuming that to 4, then when you count to four, hold your breath for 5-6 seconds and exhale slowly. Repeat this exercise 5 times - 6. Just this exercise you can do before going to bed in order to then make it easier to fall asleep.

6. "Breath" belly. The first thing to do - is to sit in a comfortable position for you. Straighten your back and lift the chin slightly up. Make a slow full breath through the nose so that the first air-filled stomach and then the chest. Briefly hold your breath. Next is to first exhale relax and lower your chest, and then gently draw the

stomach. Perform 10-15 cycles, while being careful to do as far as possible breath.

7. Inhale and exhale through different nostrils. Adopt a relaxed posture for you and close your eyes. This exercise is very simple. Plug the thumb left nostril and inhale through the right, hold your breath and exhale through the left plugged with the right nostril. Then keep your right nostril closed and inhale through the left nostril. Inhale through the left nostril, exhale through the right nostril make closing with the left nostril. Repeat this exercise several times. It is not recommended to do this exercise before bedtime.

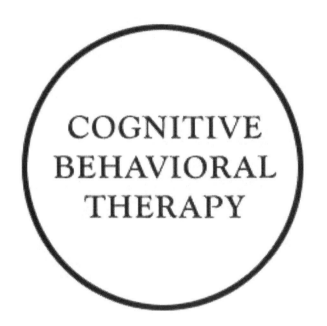

4. Exercises Based on Techniques of Psych Synthesis, Assagioli developed..

4.1. Exercise "self-correcting behavior by self-analysis" (on D. Reyuorter)

Focus on your body.

- Check all your physical sensations experienced. Note, for example, that you feel when you touch the chair you are sitting, your feet rest on the floor, in what position are your hands.

- Identify areas in which you are experiencing stress or discomfort, but do not do anything to relieve these feelings.

- Observe your breathing.

When you feel that it is enough to focus on the body, go to the next step. Following the procedure of psych synthesis to do this to impress me: "I have a body, but I - it's not the body."

Now focus on your feelings. Your goal - to remain an outside observer himself, therefore, aware of their feelings, you should stand idly by them, not to sink into their experience.

- Ask yourself, which of these feelings you experience in life more often. What are the positive and negative aspects of these feelings? When you're ready to move on, you tell yourself: "I have a feeling, but I - it's not the feelings."

Turn attention to their desires.

- List the main aspirations that drive you in life, treating them as neutral as before to the senses. Instead of thinking about the importance to you of each of them, just look at them one by one, and when you are ready, on the "five say to yourself:" I have the desire, but I - it does not desire. "

Now it's time to go to the thoughts.

- Observe how one thought comes to mind, and then gives way to another. Do not worry about the fact that you are doing something wrong. Even if you think that you have no thoughts, then it is thought - and watch her. In conclusion, exercise tell yourself: "I have thoughts, but I - this is not thought" (on D. Reyuoter).

4.2. Exercise "Who – I?" (By T. Youmens).

Select a place where no one will disturb you. Take a sheet of paper, put the date at the top and write: "Who am I?". Below, write down your answer to this question: the answer should be more open and honest as possible. Then, making periodic breaks, continue to mentally ask yourself this question and record the answers.

Sit down and relax. Close your eyes. Try not to think about anything. Again, ask yourself the question: "Who am I?" and try to grasp the answer in the form of a mental image. Do not think or talk about it, let the image to appear in the mind. Then open your eyes and how to detail describe the image; also indicate what feelings you have in connection with any and what it matters to you.

Stand so that you had some space to move. Close your eyes and ask yourself again: "Who am I?" This time, look for the answer in the movement of his body. Trust his wisdom, and let the movement itself developed as long as you do not feel that it was completed.

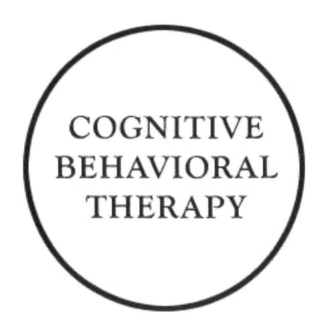

5. Exercise Emergency Psychological Self-Help ("The mental dialogue with the mirror").

Retire 10-15 minutes.

- Adopt a comfortable position, close your eyes and try to visualize yourself from the side - like his own reflection in the mirror. (It is important to notice how experienced you are currently unpleasant emotions are reflected in your mind's representation of itself - the image of "I" - on facial expressions and other features of appearance).

- Bring attention to bodily sensations and find among them those manifestations of physical discomfort that are associated with experiencing emotional discomfort.

- Mentally, referring to an imaginary reflection in the mirror as an interlocutor - about the same as the children interact with their toys - say to myself, those unsaid words in real life that you actually want to hear in your address. This may be a recognition of your rightness, praise in your address, or the compliments of comfort - in short, all that tells you the intuition - that should your sincere belief calm you, to cheer, to stop the obsessive regret and self-blame and recover your dignity; invest in them so much feeling, so much emotional pressure as if you wanted to bring your words to a real interlocutor; mental image of "I" - your imaginary interlocutor - will serve as a sensitive indicator of its "response" will show whether your words have reached the goal.

- Once again, turn your attention to bodily sensations associated with emotions. (If the eye respond to your mental dialogue, the physiological manifestations of negative emotions will also begin to subside).

Repeat these steps several times, as long as there will not disappear all manifestations of emotional bodily discomfort.

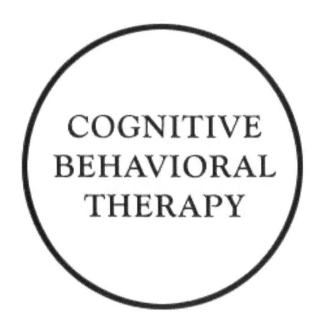

6. Exercise for "Recharging Cyanogenic Dominant" (therapeutic and supportive exercise applied after the "coding").

- Relax, sitting on a chair in a quiet secluded place with your eyes closed.

- Figuratively imagine therapist created "dominant health, recovery" - psycho-energetic source generates healing bioelectrical (preferably with the help of a doctor that "dominant" to portray, draw).

- To make a point self-massage on the forehead, said psychotherapist. Imagine if this process of development of biotite, directed to "the dominant healing" for it's charging, improve psycho-energetic potential.

- Accompany psycho-energetic self-massage targeted formulas beliefs (pronounce them better in a whisper). For example, after "coding" for alcoholism, it is recommended to say:

"I - man, divine creation of nature, and not a slave to the bottle - weapons of Satan.

I - a real man, not a limp creature.

Let punish me destiny, if I commit sin, break an oath (signature ...).

I am proud of the manifested will be coded and support (if necessary) of its healing, about alcohol effects.

Once again, I deserve respect and love...

I (name) - well, I manage myself."

My motto is:

"I - a reasonable person, not an enemy to your health and happiness"

"No I will not go astray sobriety" or

"I feel their superiority over those who continue to drink"

"I was a spiritual awakening."

Read the exercise repeatedly, until it creates a smile and a confident sense of confidence. Be healthy!

Conclusion

Several studies have examined the effectiveness of cognitive therapy, depending on the type of coping strategies and styles and customer protection. Externalities depressive patients showed better results in cognitive therapy; internality patients more supportive therapy shows where an active role in the healing of the patient plays. Over the sensitive to the cognitive impact and were less protected patients. The authors conclude that, firstly, it is necessary to take into account the psychological type of the customer's identity when choosing the type of treatment and, secondly, that cognitive therapy is indicated for the externalities and defenseless (low-resistance potential) customers.

Colleagues believe that in the next 5 years will see an incredible increase in the proportion of cognitive therapy in the overall structure of psychotherapeutic care. For cognitive therapy, they see the growing popularity of its integrative (eclectic) and empiricism (scientific nature). The strength of cognitive therapy is that it does not fight "for the purity of rows" and ready to interpenetration with other approaches.

Author

My name is Jack Oliver and me the goal is to make your life easier in the perception. All you need is knowledge that will help you get out of a stressful and depressing situation. I like to help people. I hope my work was not in vain.

P.S. You need to be patient, to go the way of healing with maximum efficiency.

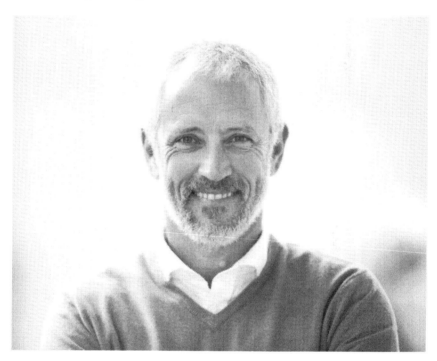

Made in the USA
Lexington, KY
01 October 2016